THIS 9
TAI CHI DAILY
JOURNAL
BELONGS TO:

_____

_____

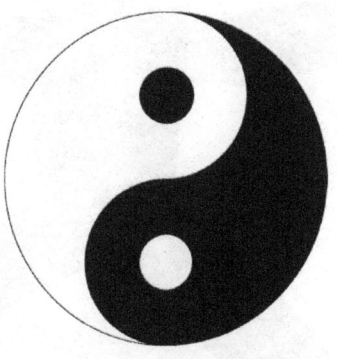

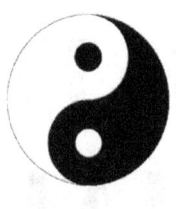

A grateful heart always makes your dreams come true.

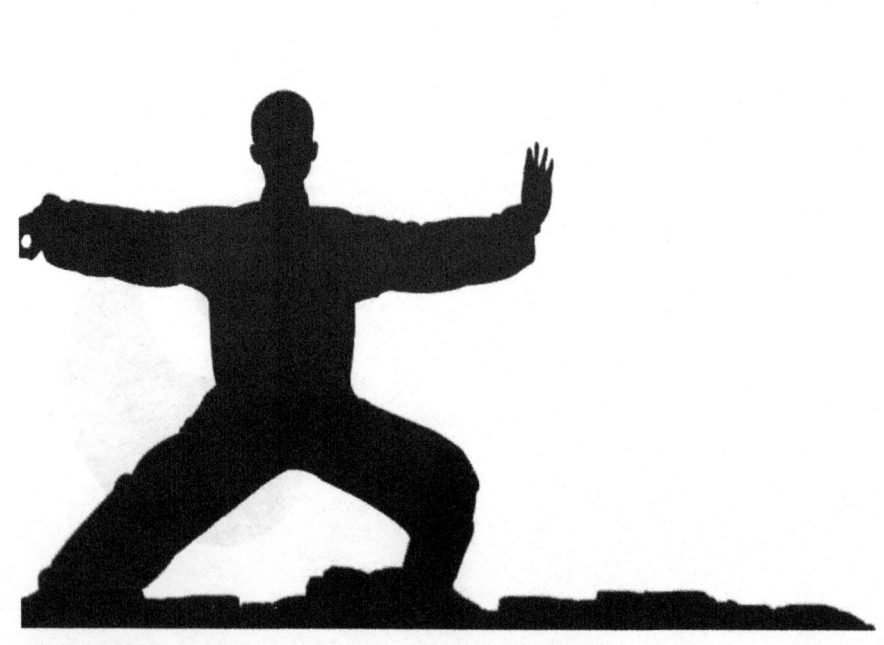

DATE: _____

| M | T | W | T | F | S | S |

Today's Intention:
_____
_____
_____

Mood:
- ❏ Fabulous
- ❏ Happy
- ❏ Sad
- ❏ Angry

Things I am Grateful For Today:
_____
_____
_____

Which forms you have exercised for today?
_____
_____

What do you like/learn during today's exercise?
_____
_____

What would you like to be improved Next time?
_____
_____

Did you feel that your health has improved? Did you feel more energetic?
_____
_____

Reviews of Exercise:

Duration:

Calories Burned:

Rating:
☆ ☆ ☆ ☆ ☆

DATE: _____

| M | T | W | T | F | S | S |

Today's Intention:
_____
_____
_____

Mood:
- ❏ Fabulous
- ❏ Happy
- ❏ Sad
- ❏ Angry

Things I am Grateful For Today:
_____
_____
_____

Which forms you have exercised for today?
_____
_____

What do you like/learn during today's exercise?
_____
_____

What would you like to be improved Next time?
_____
_____

Did you feel that your health has improved? Did you feel more energetic?
_____

Reviews of Exercise:

Duration:
Calories Burned:
Rating:
☆☆☆☆☆

DATE: _____

| M | T | W | T | F | S | S |

Today's Intention:
_____
_____
_____

Mood:
- ❑ Fabulous
- ❑ Happy
- ❑ Sad
- ❑ Angry

Things I am Grateful For Today:
_____
_____
_____

Which forms you have exercised for today?
_____
_____

What do you like/learn during today's exercise?
_____
_____

What would you like to be improved Next time?
_____
_____

Did you feel that your health has improved? Did you feel more energetic?
_____
_____

Reviews of Exercise:

Duration:

Calories Burned:

Rating:
☆ ☆ ☆ ☆ ☆

DATE: _____

| M | T | W | T | F | S | S |

TODAY'S INTENTION:
_____
_____
_____

MOOD:
- ❏ FABULOUS
- ❏ HAPPY
- ❏ SAD
- ❏ ANGRY

THINGS I AM GRATEFUL FOR TODAY:
_____
_____
_____

WHICH FORMS YOU HAVE EXERCISED FOR TODAY?
_____
_____

WHAT DO YOU LIKE/LEARN DURING TODAY'S EXERCISE?
_____
_____

WHAT WOULD YOU LIKE TO BE IMPROVED NEXT TIME?
_____
_____

DID YOU FEEL THAT YOUR HEALTH HAS IMPROVED? DID YOU FEEL MORE ENERGETIC?
_____
_____

REVIEWS OF EXERCISE:

DURATION:

CALORIES BURNED:

RATING:
☆☆☆☆☆

DATE: _____

M	T	W	T	F	S	S

TODAY'S INTENTION:
_____
_____
_____

MOOD:
- ❑ FABULOUS
- ❑ HAPPY
- ❑ SAD
- ❑ ANGRY

THINGS I AM GRATEFUL FOR TODAY:
_____
_____
_____

WHICH FORMS YOU HAVE EXERCISED FOR TODAY?
_____
_____

WHAT DO YOU LIKE/LEARN DURING TODAY'S EXERCISE?
_____
_____

WHAT WOULD YOU LIKE TO BE IMPROVED NEXT TIME?
_____
_____

DID YOU FEEL THAT YOUR HEALTH HAS IMPROVED? DID YOU FEEL MORE ENERGETIC?
_____
_____

REVIEWS OF EXERCISE:

DURATION:

CALORIES BURNED:

RATING:
★★★★☆

DATE: _____

| M | T | W | T | F | S | S |

TODAY'S INTENTION:
_____
_____
_____

MOOD:
- ❏ FABULOUS
- ❏ HAPPY
- ❏ SAD
- ❏ ANGRY

THINGS I AM GRATEFUL FOR TODAY:
_____
_____
_____

WHICH FORMS YOU HAVE EXERCISED FOR TODAY?
_____
_____

WHAT DO YOU LIKE/LEARN DURING TODAY'S EXERCISE?
_____
_____

WHAT WOULD YOU LIKE TO BE IMPROVED NEXT TIME?
_____
_____

DID YOU FEEL THAT YOUR HEALTH HAS IMPROVED? DID YOU FEEL MORE ENERGETIC?
_____

REVIEWS OF EXERCISE:

DURATION:

CALORIES BURNED:

RATING:
☆ ☆ ☆ ☆ ☆

DATE: _____

| M | T | W | T | F | S | S |

TODAY'S INTENTION:

_____
_____
_____

MOOD:
- ❑ FABULOUS
- ❑ HAPPY
- ❑ SAD
- ❑ ANGRY

THINGS I AM GRATEFUL FOR TODAY:

_____
_____
_____

WHICH FORMS YOU HAVE EXERCISED FOR TODAY?

_____
_____

WHAT DO YOU LIKE/LEARN DURING TODAY'S EXERCISE?

_____
_____

WHAT WOULD YOU LIKE TO BE IMPROVED NEXT TIME?

_____
_____

DID YOU FEEL THAT YOUR HEALTH HAS IMPROVED? DID YOU FEEL MORE ENERGETIC?

_____
_____

REVIEWS OF EXERCISE:

DURATION:

CALORIES BURNED:

RATING: ☆☆☆☆☆

DATE: _____

| M | T | W | T | F | S | S |

Today's Intention:
_____
_____
_____

MOOD:
- ❑ Fabulous
- ❑ Happy
- ❑ Sad
- ❑ Angry

Things I am Grateful For Today:
_____
_____
_____

Which forms you have exercised for today?
_____
_____

What do you like/learn during today's exercise?
_____
_____

What would you like to be improved Next time?
_____
_____

Did you feel that your health has improved? Did you feel more energetic?
_____

REVIEWS OF Exercise:

Duration:

Calories Burned:

Rating:
☆☆☆☆☆

DATE: _____

M	T	W	T	F	S	S

Today's Intention:
_____
_____
_____

MOOD:
- ❑ Fabulous
- ❑ Happy
- ❑ Sad
- ❑ Angry

Things I am Grateful For Today:
_____
_____
_____

Which forms you have exercised for today?
_____
_____

What do you like/learn during today's exercise?
_____
_____

What would you like to be improved Next time?
_____
_____

Did you feel that your health has improved? Did you feel more energetic?
_____
_____

REVIEWS OF Exercise:

Duration:

Calories Burned:

Rating:
☆☆☆☆☆

DATE: _____

| M | T | W | T | F | S | S |

Today's Intention:
_____
_____
_____

Mood:
- ❑ Fabulous
- ❑ Happy
- ❑ Sad
- ❑ Angry

Things I am Grateful For Today:
_____
_____
_____

Which forms you have exercised for today?
_____
_____

What do you like/learn during today's exercise?
_____
_____

What would you like to be improved Next time?
_____
_____

Did you feel that your health has improved? Did you feel more energetic?
_____
_____

Reviews of Exercise:

Duration:

Calories Burned:

Rating:
☆☆☆☆☆

Review

Review your experience with the past 10 days of your tai chi journey. Put down plans for the next 10 days.

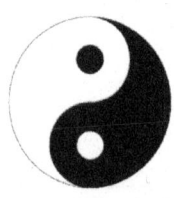

~ Gratitude cures your mind, body & heart.~

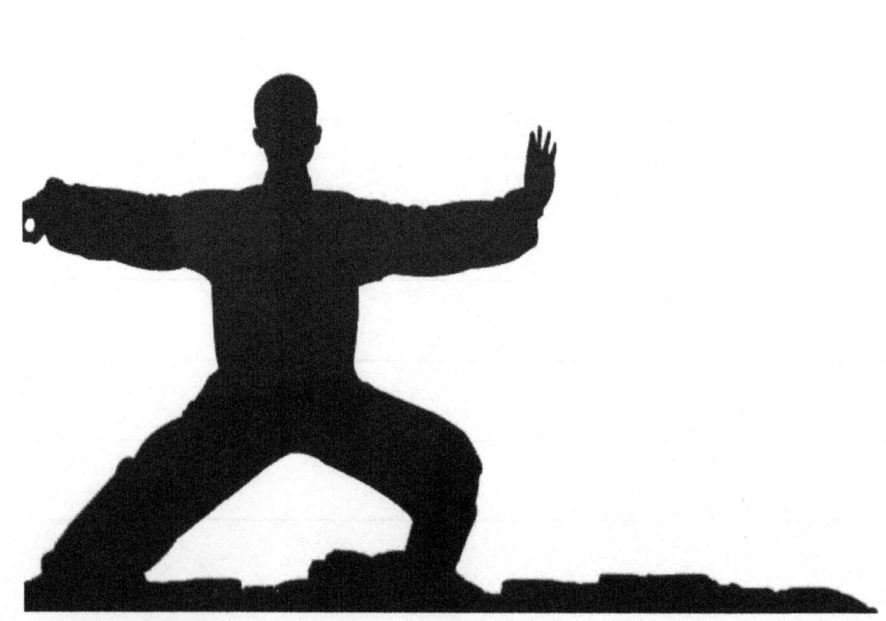

DATE: _____

| M | T | W | T | F | S | S |

Today's Intention:
_____
_____
_____

Mood:
- ❏ Fabulous
- ❏ Happy
- ❏ Sad
- ❏ Angry

Things I am Grateful For Today:
_____
_____
_____

Which forms you have exercised for today?
_____
_____

What do you like/learn during today's exercise?
_____
_____

What would you like to be improved Next time?
_____
_____

Did you feel that your health has improved? Did you feel more energetic?
_____
_____

Reviews of Exercise:

Duration:

Calories Burned:

Rating:
☆☆☆☆☆

DATE: _____

| M | T | W | T | F | S | S |

TODAY'S INTENTION:
_____
_____
_____

MOOD:
- ☐ FABULOUS
- ☐ HAPPY
- ☐ SAD
- ☐ ANGRY

THINGS I AM GRATEFUL FOR TODAY:
_____
_____
_____

WHICH FORMS YOU HAVE EXERCISED FOR TODAY?
_____
_____

WHAT DO YOU LIKE/LEARN DURING TODAY'S EXERCISE?
_____
_____

WHAT WOULD YOU LIKE TO BE IMPROVED NEXT TIME?
_____
_____

DID YOU FEEL THAT YOUR HEALTH HAS IMPROVED? DID YOU FEEL MORE ENERGETIC?
_____
_____

REVIEWS OF EXERCISE:

DURATION:

CALORIES BURNED:

RATING:
★☆☆☆☆

DATE: _____

| M | T | W | T | F | S | S |

Today's Intention:
_____
_____
_____

Mood:
- ❑ Fabulous
- ❑ Happy
- ❑ Sad
- ❑ Angry

Things I am Grateful For Today:
_____
_____
_____

Which forms you have exercised for today?
_____
_____

What do you like/learn during today's exercise?
_____
_____

What would you like to be improved Next time?
_____
_____

Did you feel that your health has improved? Did you feel more energetic?
_____
_____

Reviews of Exercise:

Duration:

Calories Burned:

Rating:
☆☆☆☆☆

DATE: _____

| M | T | W | T | F | S | S |

Today's Intention:
_____
_____
_____

MOOD:
- ❏ Fabulous
- ❏ Happy
- ❏ Sad
- ❏ Angry

Things I am Grateful For Today:
_____
_____
_____

Which forms you have exercised for today?
_____
_____

What do you like/learn during today's exercise?
_____
_____

What would you like to be improved Next time?
_____
_____

Did you feel that your health has improved? Did you feel more energetic?
_____
_____

Reviews of Exercise:

Duration:

Calories Burned:

Rating: ☆☆☆☆☆

DATE: _____

| M | T | W | T | F | S | S |

TODAY'S INTENTION:
_____
_____
_____

MOOD:
- ❏ FABULOUS
- ❏ HAPPY
- ❏ SAD
- ❏ ANGRY

THINGS I AM GRATEFUL FOR TODAY:
_____
_____
_____

WHICH FORMS YOU HAVE EXERCISED FOR TODAY?
_____
_____

WHAT DO YOU LIKE/LEARN DURING TODAY'S EXERCISE?
_____
_____

WHAT WOULD YOU LIKE TO BE IMPROVED NEXT TIME?
_____
_____

DID YOU FEEL THAT YOUR HEALTH HAS IMPROVED? DID YOU FEEL MORE ENERGETIC?
_____
_____

REVIEWS OF EXERCISE:

DURATION:

CALORIES BURNED:

RATING:
☆☆☆☆☆

DATE: _____

| M | T | W | T | F | S | S |

TODAY'S INTENTION:
_____
_____
_____

MOOD:
- ❑ FABULOUS
- ❑ HAPPY
- ❑ SAD
- ❑ ANGRY

THINGS I AM GRATEFUL FOR TODAY:
_____
_____
_____

WHICH FORMS YOU HAVE EXERCISED FOR TODAY?
_____
_____

WHAT DO YOU LIKE/LEARN DURING TODAY'S EXERCISE?
_____
_____

WHAT WOULD YOU LIKE TO BE IMPROVED NEXT TIME?
_____
_____

DID YOU FEEL THAT YOUR HEALTH HAS IMPROVED? DID YOU FEEL MORE ENERGETIC?
_____
_____

REVIEWS OF EXERCISE:

DURATION:

CALORIES BURNED:

RATING:
☆ ☆ ☆ ☆ ☆

DATE: _____

| M | T | W | T | F | S | S |

TODAY'S INTENTION:
_____
_____
_____

MOOD:
- ❑ FABULOUS
- ❑ HAPPY
- ❑ SAD
- ❑ ANGRY

THINGS I AM GRATEFUL FOR TODAY:
_____
_____
_____

WHICH FORMS YOU HAVE EXERCISED FOR TODAY?
_____
_____

WHAT DO YOU LIKE/LEARN DURING TODAY'S EXERCISE?
_____
_____

WHAT WOULD YOU LIKE TO BE IMPROVED NEXT TIME?
_____
_____

DID YOU FEEL THAT YOUR HEALTH HAS IMPROVED? DID YOU FEEL MORE ENERGETIC?
_____
_____

REVIEWS OF EXERCISE:

DURATION:

CALORIES BURNED:

RATING:
☆ ☆ ☆ ☆ ☆

DATE: _____

| M | T | W | T | F | S | S |

Today's Intention:
_____
_____
_____

MOOD:
- ❑ Fabulous
- ❑ Happy
- ❑ Sad
- ❑ Angry

Things I am Grateful For Today:
_____
_____
_____

Which forms you have exercised for today?
_____
_____

What do you like/learn during today's exercise?
_____
_____

What would you like to be improved Next time?
_____
_____

Did you feel that your health has improved? Did you feel more energetic?
_____
_____

Reviews of Exercise:

Duration:

Calories Burned:

Rating: ☆☆☆☆☆

DATE: _____

| M | T | W | T | F | S | S |

TODAY'S INTENTION:
_____
_____
_____

MOOD:
- ❑ FABULOUS
- ❑ HAPPY
- ❑ SAD
- ❑ ANGRY

THINGS I AM GRATEFUL FOR TODAY:
_____
_____
_____

WHICH FORMS YOU HAVE EXERCISED FOR TODAY?
_____
_____

WHAT DO YOU LIKE/LEARN DURING TODAY'S EXERCISE?
_____
_____

WHAT WOULD YOU LIKE TO BE IMPROVED NEXT TIME?
_____
_____

DID YOU FEEL THAT YOUR HEALTH HAS IMPROVED? DID YOU FEEL MORE ENERGETIC?
_____
_____

REVIEWS OF EXERCISE:

DURATION:

CALORIES BURNED:

RATING:
☆☆☆☆☆

DATE: _____

| M | T | W | T | F | S | S |

TODAY'S INTENTION:
_____
_____
_____

MOOD:
- ❏ FABULOUS
- ❏ HAPPY
- ❏ SAD
- ❏ ANGRY

THINGS I AM GRATEFUL FOR TODAY:
_____
_____
_____

WHICH FORMS YOU HAVE EXERCISED FOR TODAY?
_____
_____

WHAT DO YOU LIKE/LEARN DURING TODAY'S EXERCISE?
_____
_____

WHAT WOULD YOU LIKE TO BE IMPROVED NEXT TIME?
_____
_____

DID YOU FEEL THAT YOUR HEALTH HAS IMPROVED? DID YOU FEEL MORE ENERGETIC?
_____
_____

REVIEWS OF EXERCISE:

DURATION:

CALORIES BURNED:

RATING:
☆☆☆☆☆

REVIEW

REVIEW YOUR EXPERIENCE WITH THE PAST 10 DAYS OF YOUR TAI CHI JOURNEY. PUT DOWN PLANS FOR THE NEXT 10 DAYS.

_____
_____
_____
_____
_____
_____
_____
_____
_____
_____
_____
_____
_____
_____
_____
_____
_____
_____

Gratitude is a magnet for more stuff that you would be grateful for

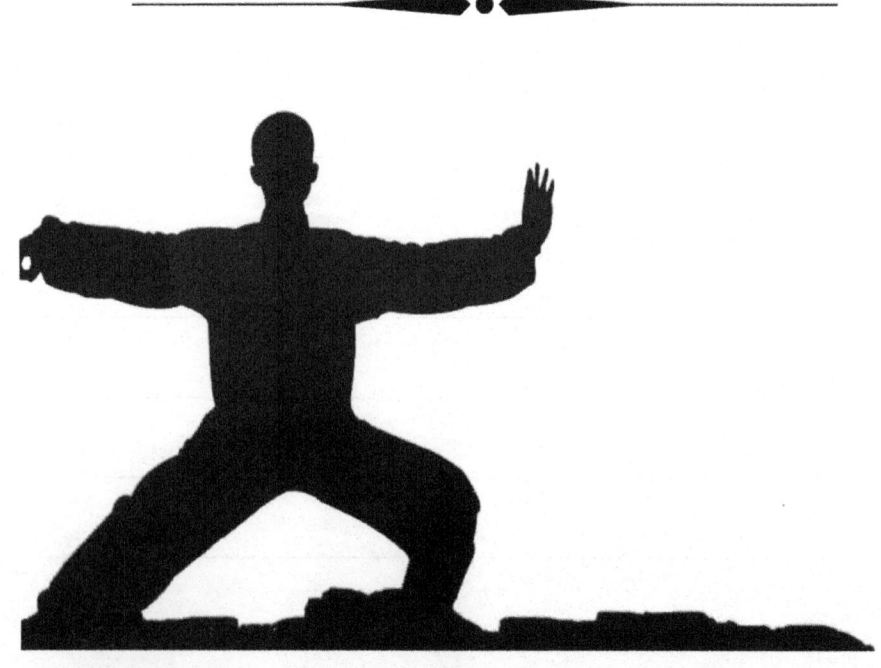

DATE: _____

| M | T | W | T | F | S | S |

Today's Intention:
_____
_____
_____

MOOD:
- ❏ Fabulous
- ❏ Happy
- ❏ Sad
- ❏ Angry

Things I am Grateful For Today:
_____
_____
_____

Which forms you have exercised for today?
_____
_____

What do you like/learn during today's exercise?
_____
_____

What would you like to be improved Next time?
_____
_____

Did you feel that your health has improved? Did you feel more energetic?
_____
_____

REVIEWS OF Exercise:

Duration:

Calories Burned:

Rating:
★★★★☆

DATE: _____

| M | T | W | T | F | S | S |

Today's Intention:
_____
_____
_____

Mood:
- ❏ Fabulous
- ❏ Happy
- ❏ Sad
- ❏ Angry

Things I am Grateful For Today:
_____
_____
_____

Which forms you have exercised for today?
_____
_____

What do you like/learn during today's exercise?
_____
_____

What would you like to be improved Next time?
_____
_____

Did you feel that your health has improved? Did you feel more energetic?
_____
_____

Reviews of Exercise:

Duration:

Calories Burned:

Rating:
☆☆☆☆☆

DATE: _____

| M | T | W | T | F | S | S |

Today's Intention:
_____
_____
_____

MOOD:
- ❑ Fabulous
- ❑ Happy
- ❑ Sad
- ❑ Angry

Things I am Grateful For Today:
_____
_____
_____

Which forms you have exercised for today?
_____
_____

What do you like/learn during today's exercise?
_____
_____

What would you like to be improved Next time?
_____
_____

Did you feel that your health has improved? Did you feel more energetic?
_____
_____

REVIEWS OF Exercise:

Duration:

Calories Burned:

Rating:
☆☆☆☆☆

DATE: _____

M	T	W	T	F	S	S

Today's Intention:
_____
_____
_____

MOOD:
- ❏ Fabulous
- ❏ Happy
- ❏ Sad
- ❏ Angry

Things I am Grateful For Today:
_____
_____
_____

Which forms you have exercised for today?
_____
_____

What do you like/learn during today's exercise?
_____
_____

What would you like to be improved Next time?
_____
_____

Did you feel that your health has improved? Did you feel more energetic?
_____

Reviews of Exercise:

Duration:

Calories Burned:

Rating:
☆☆☆☆☆

DATE: _____

Today's Intention:
_____
_____
_____

| M | T | W | T | F | S | S |

MOOD:
- ❏ Fabulous
- ❏ Happy
- ❏ Sad
- ❏ Angry

Things I am Grateful For Today:
_____
_____

Which forms you have exercised for today?
_____
_____

What do you like/learn during today's exercise?
_____
_____

What would you like to be improved next time?
_____
_____

Did you feel that your health has improved? Did you feel more energetic?
_____
_____

Reviews of Exercise:

Duration:

Calories Burned:

Rating:
☆☆☆☆☆

DATE: _____

| M | T | W | T | F | S | S |

Today's Intention:
_____
_____
_____

Mood:
- ❑ Fabulous
- ❑ Happy
- ❑ Sad
- ❑ Angry

Things I am Grateful For Today:
_____
_____
_____

Which forms you have exercised for today?
_____
_____

What do you like/learn during today's exercise?
_____
_____

What would you like to be improved Next time?
_____
_____

Did you feel that your health has improved? Did you feel more energetic?
_____
_____

Reviews of Exercise:

Duration:

Calories Burned:

Rating:
☆☆☆☆☆

DATE: _____

M	T	W	T	F	S	S

Today's Intention:
_____
_____
_____

Mood:
- ❏ Fabulous
- ❏ Happy
- ❏ Sad
- ❏ Angry

Things I am Grateful For Today:
_____
_____
_____

Which forms you have exercised for today?
_____
_____

What do you like/learn during today's exercise?
_____
_____

What would you like to be improved Next time?
_____
_____

Did you feel that your health has improved? Did you feel more energetic?
_____
_____

Reviews of Exercise:

Duration:

Calories Burned:

Rating:
☆☆☆☆☆

DATE: _____

| M | T | W | T | F | S | S |

Today's Intention:
_____
_____
_____

MOOD:
☐ Fabulous
☐ Happy
☐ Sad
☐ Angry

Things I am Grateful For Today:
_____
_____
_____

Which forms you have exercised for today?
_____
_____

What do you like/learn during today's exercise?
_____
_____

What would you like to be improved Next time?
_____
_____

Did you feel that your health has improved? Did you feel more energetic?
_____
_____

Reviews of Exercise:

Duration:

Calories Burned:

Rating:
☆☆☆☆☆

DATE: _____

| M | T | W | T | F | S | S |

Today's Intention:
_____
_____
_____

MOOD:
- ❏ Fabulous
- ❏ Happy
- ❏ Sad
- ❏ Angry

Things I am Grateful For Today:
_____
_____
_____

Which forms you have exercised for today?
_____
_____

What do you like/learn during today's exercise?
_____
_____

What would you like to be improved Next time?
_____
_____

Did you feel that your health has improved? Did you feel more energetic?
_____
_____

REVIEWS OF Exercise:

Duration:

Calories Burned:

Rating:
☆☆☆☆☆

DATE: _____

M	T	W	T	F	S	S

Today's Intention:
_____
_____
_____

MOOD:
- ❑ Fabulous
- ❑ Happy
- ❑ Sad
- ❑ Angry

Things I am Grateful For Today:
_____
_____
_____

Which forms you have exercised for today?
_____
_____

What do you like/learn during today's exercise?
_____
_____

What would you like to be improved Next time?
_____
_____

Did you feel that your health has improved? Did you feel more energetic?
_____
_____

REVIEWS OF EXERCISE:

DURATION:

CALORIES BURNED:

RATING:
☆☆☆☆☆

Review

Review your experience with the past 10 days of your tai chi journey. Put down plans for the next 10 days.

_____
_____
_____
_____
_____
_____
_____
_____
_____
_____
_____
_____
_____
_____
_____
_____
_____

Gratitude is the best supplement for your health.

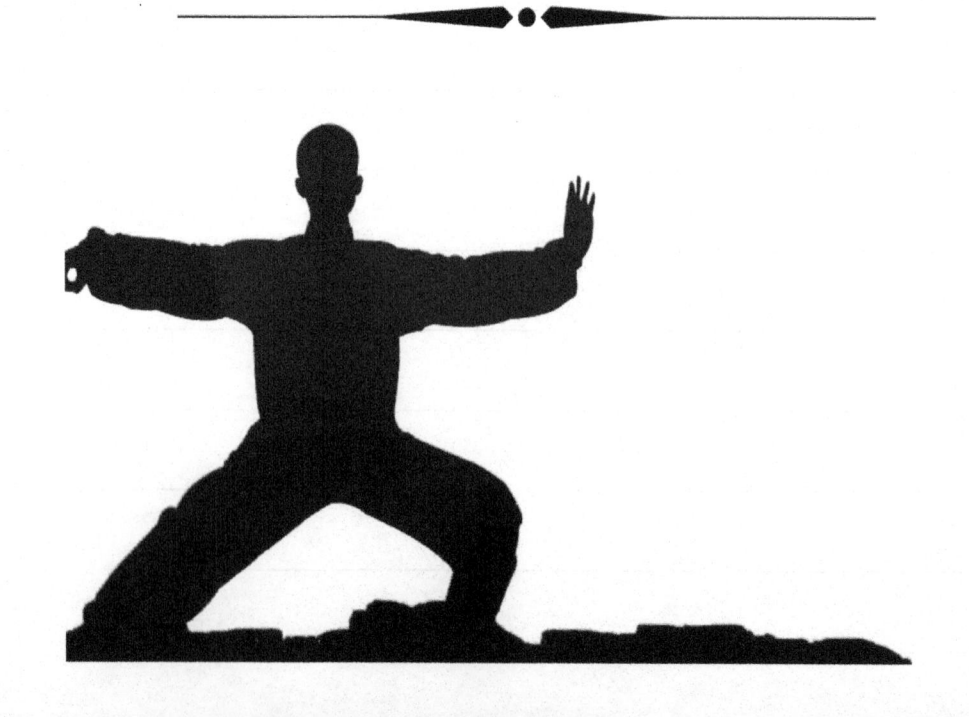

DATE: _____

| M | T | W | T | F | S | S |

Today's Intention:
_____
_____
_____

MOOD:
❑ Fabulous
❑ Happy
❑ Sad
❑ Angry

Things I am Grateful For Today:
_____
_____
_____
_____

Which forms you have exercised for today?
_____
_____

What do you like/learn during today's exercise?
_____
_____

What would you like to be improved Next time?
_____
_____

Did you feel that your health has improved? Did you feel more energetic?
_____
_____

REVIEWS OF Exercise:

Duration:

Calories Burned:

Rating:
☆ ☆ ☆ ☆ ☆

DATE: _____

M	T	W	T	F	S	S

Today's Intention:
_____
_____
_____

MOOD:
- ❏ Fabulous
- ❏ Happy
- ❏ Sad
- ❏ Angry

Things I am Grateful For Today:
_____
_____
_____

Which forms you have exercised for today?
_____
_____

What do you like/learn during today's exercise?
_____
_____

What would you like to be improved Next time?
_____
_____

Did you feel that your health has improved? Did you feel more energetic?
_____
_____

REVIEWS OF EXERCISE:

DURATION:

CALORIES BURNED:

RATING:
☆☆☆☆☆

DATE: _____

| M | T | W | T | F | S | S |

Today's Intention:
_____
_____
_____

MOOD:
- ❏ Fabulous
- ❏ Happy
- ❏ Sad
- ❏ Angry

Things I am Grateful For Today:
_____
_____
_____

Which forms you have exercised for today?
_____
_____

What do you like/learn during today's exercise?
_____
_____

What would you like to be improved Next time?
_____
_____

Did you feel that your health has improved? Did you feel more energetic?
_____

Reviews of Exercise:

Duration:

Calories Burned:

Rating:
☆☆☆☆☆

DATE: _____

| M | T | W | T | F | S | S |

TODAY'S INTENTION:
_____
_____
_____

MOOD:
- ❏ FABULOUS
- ❏ HAPPY
- ❏ SAD
- ❏ ANGRY

THINGS I AM GRATEFUL FOR TODAY:
_____
_____
_____

WHICH FORMS YOU HAVE EXERCISED FOR TODAY?
_____
_____

WHAT DO YOU LIKE/LEARN DURING TODAY'S EXERCISE?
_____
_____

WHAT WOULD YOU LIKE TO BE IMPROVED NEXT TIME?
_____
_____

DID YOU FEEL THAT YOUR HEALTH HAS IMPROVED? DID YOU FEEL MORE ENERGETIC?
_____
_____

REVIEWS OF EXERCISE:

DURATION:

CALORIES BURNED:

RATING:
☆☆☆☆☆

DATE: _____

M	T	W	T	F	S	S

Today's Intention:
_____
_____
_____

MOOD:
❏ Fabulous
❏ Happy
❏ Sad
❏ Angry

Things I am Grateful For Today:
_____
_____
_____

Which forms you have exercised for today?
_____
_____

What do you like/learn during today's exercise?
_____
_____

What would you like to be improved Next time?
_____
_____

Did you feel that your health has improved? Did you feel more energetic?
_____
_____

REVIEWS OF Exercise:

Duration:

Calories Burned:

Rating:
★★★★☆

DATE: _____

| M | T | W | T | F | S | S |

Today's Intention:
_____
_____
_____

MOOD:
- ❑ Fabulous
- ❑ Happy
- ❑ Sad
- ❑ Angry

Things I am Grateful For Today:
_____
_____
_____

Which forms you have exercised for today?
_____
_____

What do you like/learn during today's exercise?
_____
_____

What would you like to be improved Next time?
_____
_____

Did you feel that your health has improved? Did you feel more energetic?
_____
_____

REVIEWS OF Exercise:

Duration:

Calories Burned:

Rating:
☆☆☆☆☆

DATE: _____

Today's Intention:
_____
_____
_____

| M | T | W | T | F | S | S |

MOOD:
- ❏ Fabulous
- ❏ Happy
- ❏ Sad
- ❏ Angry

Things I Am Grateful For Today:
_____
_____
_____

Which forms you have exercised for today?
_____
_____

What do you like/learn during today's exercise?
_____
_____

What would you like to be improved next time?
_____
_____

Did you feel that your health has improved? Did you feel more energetic?
_____
_____

REVIEWS OF EXERCISE:

DURATION:

CALORIES BURNED:

RATING:
☆ ☆ ☆ ☆ ☆

DATE: _____

| M | T | W | T | F | S | S |

Today's Intention:
_____
_____
_____

MOOD:
- ❑ Fabulous
- ❑ Happy
- ❑ Sad
- ❑ Angry

Things I am Grateful For Today:
_____
_____
_____

Which forms you have exercised for today?
_____
_____

What do you like/learn during today's exercise?
_____
_____

What would you like to be improved Next time?
_____
_____

Did you feel that your health has improved? Did you feel more energetic?
_____
_____

Reviews Of Exercise:

Duration:

Calories Burned:

Rating: ☆☆☆☆☆

DATE: _____

| M | T | W | T | F | S | S |

TODAY'S INTENTION:

_____

MOOD:
- ❏ FABULOUS
- ❏ HAPPY
- ❏ SAD
- ❏ ANGRY

THINGS I AM GRATEFUL FOR TODAY:

_____

WHICH FORMS YOU HAVE EXERCISED FOR TODAY?

_____

WHAT DO YOU LIKE/LEARN DURING TODAY'S EXERCISE?

_____

WHAT WOULD YOU LIKE TO BE IMPROVED NEXT TIME?

_____

DID YOU FEEL THAT YOUR HEALTH HAS IMPROVED? DID YOU FEEL MORE ENERGETIC?

_____

REVIEWS OF EXERCISE:

DURATION:

CALORIES BURNED:

RATING:
☆☆☆☆☆

DATE: _____

M	T	W	T	F	S	S

Today's Intention:
_____
_____
_____

MOOD:
- ❑ Fabulous
- ❑ Happy
- ❑ Sad
- ❑ Angry

Things I am Grateful For Today:
_____
_____
_____

Which forms you have exercised for today?
_____
_____

What do you like/learn during today's exercise?
_____
_____

What would you like to be improved Next time?
_____
_____

Did you feel that your health has improved? Did you feel more energetic?
_____
_____

Reviews of Exercise:

Duration:

Calories Burned:

Rating:
☆☆☆☆☆

Review

Review your experience with the past 10 days of your tai chi journey. Put down plans for the next 10 days.

_____
_____
_____
_____
_____
_____
_____
_____
_____
_____
_____
_____
_____
_____
_____
_____
_____
_____

~ Say thanks to your loved ones would make their day. ~

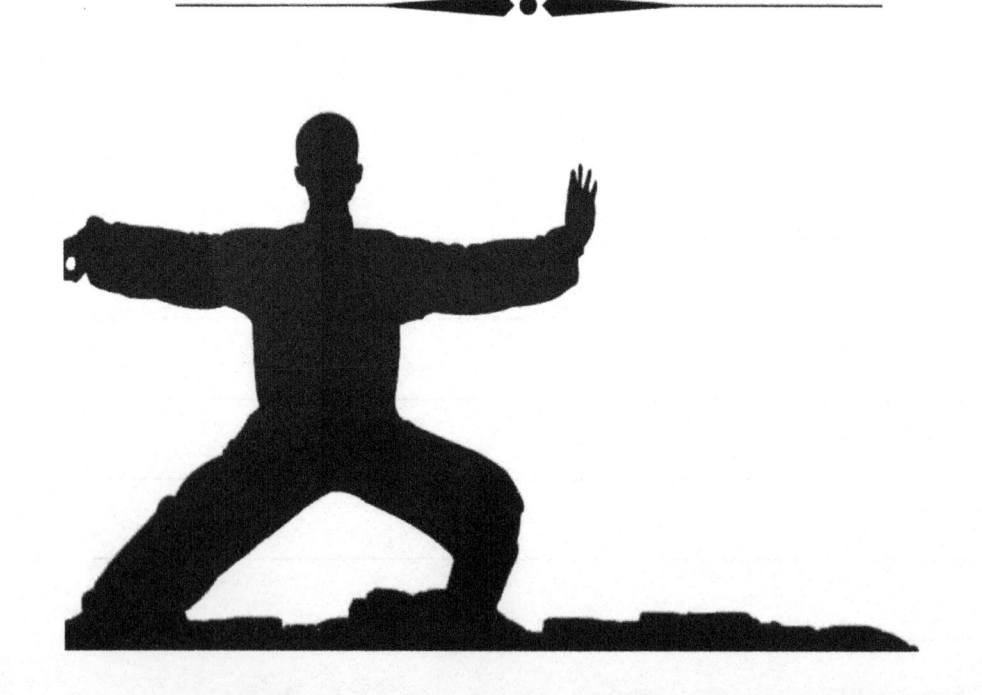

DATE: _____

| M | T | W | T | F | S | S |

TODAY'S INTENTION:
_____
_____
_____

MOOD:
- ❏ FABULOUS
- ❏ HAPPY
- ❏ SAD
- ❏ ANGRY

THINGS I AM GRATEFUL FOR TODAY:
_____
_____
_____

WHICH FORMS YOU HAVE EXERCISED FOR TODAY?
_____
_____

WHAT DO YOU LIKE/LEARN DURING TODAY'S EXERCISE?
_____
_____

WHAT WOULD YOU LIKE TO BE IMPROVED NEXT TIME?
_____
_____

DID YOU FEEL THAT YOUR HEALTH HAS IMPROVED? DID YOU FEEL MORE ENERGETIC?
_____
_____

REVIEWS OF EXERCISE:

DURATION:

CALORIES BURNED:

RATING:
☆☆☆☆☆

DATE: _____

| M | T | W | T | F | S | S |

Today's Intention:
_____
_____
_____

MOOD:
- ❏ Fabulous
- ❏ Happy
- ❏ Sad
- ❏ Angry

Things I am Grateful For Today:
_____
_____
_____

Which forms you have exercised for today?
_____
_____
_____

What do you like/learn during today's exercise?
_____
_____

What would you like to be improved Next time?
_____
_____

Did you feel that your health has improved? Did you feel more energetic?
_____
_____

Reviews of Exercise:

Duration:

Calories Burned:

Rating:
☆☆☆☆☆

DATE: _____

M	T	W	T	F	S	S

Today's Intention:
_____
_____
_____

MOOD:
- ❏ Fabulous
- ❏ Happy
- ❏ Sad
- ❏ Angry

Things I am Grateful For Today:
_____
_____
_____

Which forms you have exercised for today?
_____
_____

What do you like/learn during today's exercise?
_____
_____

What would you like to be improved Next time?
_____
_____

Did you feel that your health has improved? Did you feel more energetic?
_____

REVIEWS OF Exercise:

Duration:

Calories Burned:

Rating:
☆☆☆☆☆

DATE: _____

| M | T | W | T | F | S | S |

Today's Intention:
_____
_____
_____

MOOD:
- ❏ Fabulous
- ❏ Happy
- ❏ Sad
- ❏ Angry

Things I am Grateful For Today:
_____
_____
_____

Which forms you have exercised for today?
_____
_____

What do you like/learn during today's exercise?
_____
_____

What would you like to be improved Next time?
_____
_____

Did you feel that your health has improved? Did you feel more energetic?
_____
_____

REVIEWS OF Exercise:

Duration:

Calories Burned:

Rating:
☆☆☆☆☆

DATE: _____

| M | T | W | T | F | S | S |

Today's Intention:
_____
_____
_____

MOOD:
- ❑ Fabulous
- ❑ Happy
- ❑ Sad
- ❑ Angry

Things I am Grateful For Today:
_____
_____
_____

Which forms you have exercised for today?
_____
_____

What do you like/learn during today's exercise?
_____
_____

What would you like to be improved Next time?
_____
_____

Did you feel that your health has improved? Did you feel more energetic?
_____
_____

Reviews of Exercise:

Duration:

Calories Burned:

Rating:
★★★★☆

DATE: _____

| M | T | W | T | F | S | S |

Today's Intention:
_____
_____
_____

Mood:
- ❏ Fabulous
- ❏ Happy
- ❏ Sad
- ❏ Angry

Things I am Grateful For Today:
_____
_____
_____

Which forms you have exercised for today?
_____
_____

What do you like/learn during today's exercise?
_____
_____

What would you like to be improved Next time?
_____
_____

Did you feel that your health has improved? Did you feel more energetic?
_____
_____

Reviews of Exercise:

Duration:

Calories Burned:

Rating:
☆☆☆☆☆

DATE: _____

| M | T | W | T | F | S | S |

Today's Intention:
_____
_____
_____

MOOD:
- ❑ Fabulous
- ❑ Happy
- ❑ Sad
- ❑ Angry

Things I am Grateful For Today:
_____
_____
_____

Which forms you have exercised for today?
_____
_____

What do you like/learn during today's exercise?
_____
_____

What would you like to be improved Next time?
_____
_____

Did you feel that your health has improved? Did you feel more energetic?
_____
_____

REVIEWS OF Exercise:

Duration:

Calories Burned:

Rating:
☆☆☆☆☆

DATE: _____

| M | T | W | T | F | S | S |

TODAY'S INTENTION:
_____
_____
_____

MOOD:
- ❑ Fabulous
- ❑ Happy
- ❑ Sad
- ❑ Angry

THINGS I AM GRATEFUL FOR TODAY:
_____
_____

WHICH FORMS YOU HAVE EXERCISED FOR TODAY?
_____
_____

WHAT DO YOU LIKE/LEARN DURING TODAY'S EXERCISE?
_____
_____

WHAT WOULD YOU LIKE TO BE IMPROVED NEXT TIME?
_____
_____

DID YOU FEEL THAT YOUR HEALTH HAS IMPROVED? DID YOU FEEL MORE ENERGETIC?
_____
_____

REVIEWS OF EXERCISE:

DURATION:

CALORIES BURNED:

RATING:
☆☆☆☆☆

DATE: _____

| M | T | W | T | F | S | S |

TODAY'S INTENTION:
_____
_____
_____

MOOD:
❑ FABULOUS
❑ HAPPY
❑ SAD
❑ ANGRY

THINGS I AM GRATEFUL FOR TODAY:
_____
_____
_____

WHICH FORMS YOU HAVE EXERCISED FOR TODAY?
_____
_____

WHAT DO YOU LIKE/LEARN DURING TODAY'S EXERCISE?
_____
_____

WHAT WOULD YOU LIKE TO BE IMPROVED NEXT TIME?
_____
_____

DID YOU FEEL THAT YOUR HEALTH HAS IMPROVED? DID YOU FEEL MORE ENERGETIC?
_____
_____

REVIEWS OF EXERCISE:

DURATION:

CALORIES BURNED:

RATING:
☆☆☆☆☆

DATE: _____

| M | T | W | T | F | S | S |

Today's Intention:
_____
_____
_____

MOOD:
- ❑ Fabulous
- ❑ Happy
- ❑ Sad
- ❑ Angry

Things I am Grateful For Today:
_____
_____
_____

Which forms you have exercised for today?
_____
_____

What do you like/learn during today's exercise?
_____
_____

What would you like to be improved Next time?
_____
_____

Did you feel that your health has improved? Did you feel more energetic?
_____
_____

REVIEWS OF Exercise:

Duration:

Calories Burned:

Rating:
☆☆☆☆☆

Review

Review your experience with the past 10 days of your tai chi journey. Put down plans for the next 10 days.

_____
_____
_____
_____
_____
_____
_____
_____
_____
_____
_____
_____
_____
_____
_____
_____
_____

Take in love. Give out gratitude.

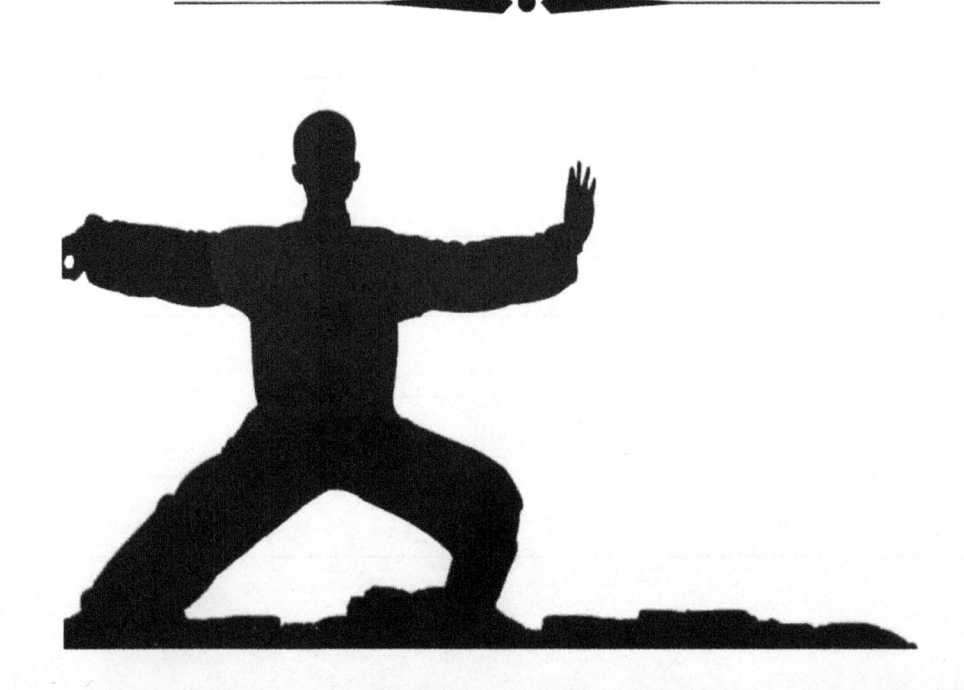

DATE: _____

| M | T | W | T | F | S | S |

TODAY'S INTENTION:
_____
_____
_____

MOOD:
- ❑ FABULOUS
- ❑ HAPPY
- ❑ SAD
- ❑ ANGRY

THINGS I AM GRATEFUL FOR TODAY:
_____
_____
_____

WHICH FORMS YOU HAVE EXERCISED FOR TODAY?
_____
_____

WHAT DO YOU LIKE/LEARN DURING TODAY'S EXERCISE?
_____
_____

WHAT WOULD YOU LIKE TO BE IMPROVED NEXT TIME?
_____
_____

DID YOU FEEL THAT YOUR HEALTH HAS IMPROVED? DID YOU FEEL MORE ENERGETIC?
_____
_____

REVIEWS OF EXERCISE:

DURATION:

CALORIES BURNED:

RATING:
☆ ☆ ☆ ☆ ☆

DATE: _____ | M | T | W | T | F | S | S |

TODAY'S INTENTION:

_____
_____
_____

MOOD:
- ❏ FABULOUS
- ❏ HAPPY
- ❏ SAD
- ❏ ANGRY

THINGS I AM GRATEFUL FOR TODAY:
_____
_____
_____

WHICH FORMS YOU HAVE EXERCISED FOR TODAY?
_____
_____

WHAT DO YOU LIKE/LEARN DURING TODAY'S EXERCISE?
_____
_____

WHAT WOULD YOU LIKE TO BE IMPROVED NEXT TIME?
_____
_____

DID YOU FEEL THAT YOUR HEALTH HAS IMPROVED? DID YOU FEEL MORE ENERGETIC?
_____

REVIEWS OF EXERCISE:

DURATION:

CALORIES BURNED:

RATING: ☆☆☆☆☆

DATE: _____

| M | T | W | T | F | S | S |

Today's Intention:
_____
_____
_____

MOOD:
- ❏ Fabulous
- ❏ Happy
- ❏ Sad
- ❏ Angry

Things I am Grateful For Today:
_____
_____
_____

Which forms you have exercised for today?
_____
_____

What do you like/learn during today's exercise?
_____
_____

What would you like to be improved Next time?
_____
_____

Did you feel that your health has improved? Did you feel more energetic?
_____
_____

REVIEWS OF Exercise:

Duration:

Calories Burned:

Rating:
☆☆☆☆☆

DATE: _____

| M | T | W | T | F | S | S |

TODAY'S INTENTION:
_____
_____
_____

MOOD:
❑ FABULOUS
❑ HAPPY
❑ SAD
❑ ANGRY

THINGS I AM GRATEFUL FOR TODAY:
_____
_____
_____

WHICH FORMS YOU HAVE EXERCISED FOR TODAY?
_____
_____

WHAT DO YOU LIKE/LEARN DURING TODAY'S EXERCISE?
_____
_____

WHAT WOULD YOU LIKE TO BE IMPROVED NEXT TIME?
_____
_____

DID YOU FEEL THAT YOUR HEALTH HAS IMPROVED? DID YOU FEEL MORE ENERGETIC?
_____
_____

REVIEWS OF EXERCISE:

DURATION:

CALORIES BURNED:

RATING:
☆☆☆☆☆

DATE: _____

| M | T | W | T | F | S | S |

Today's Intention:
_____
_____
_____

MOOD:
- ❏ Fabulous
- ❏ Happy
- ❏ Sad
- ❏ Angry

Things I am Grateful For Today:
_____
_____
_____

Which forms you have exercised for today?
_____
_____

What do you like/learn during today's exercise?
_____
_____

What would you like to be improved Next time?
_____
_____

Did you feel that your health has improved? Did you feel more energetic?
_____

Reviews of Exercise:

Duration:

Calories Burned:

Rating: ☆☆☆☆☆

DATE: _____

| M | T | W | T | F | S | S |

Today's Intention:
_____
_____
_____

MOOD:
- ❑ Fabulous
- ❑ Happy
- ❑ Sad
- ❑ Angry

Things I am Grateful For Today:
_____
_____
_____

Which forms you have exercised for today?
_____
_____

What do you like/learn during today's exercise?
_____
_____

What would you like to be improved Next time?
_____
_____

Did you feel that your health has improved? Did you feel more energetic?
_____
_____

Reviews of Exercise:

Duration:

Calories Burned:

Rating:
☆☆☆☆☆

DATE: _____

| M | T | W | T | F | S | S |

Today's Intention:
_____
_____
_____

MOOD:
- ❏ Fabulous
- ❏ Happy
- ❏ Sad
- ❏ Angry

Things I am Grateful For Today:
_____
_____
_____

Which forms you have exercised for today?
_____
_____

What do you like/learn during today's exercise?
_____
_____

What would you like to be improved Next time?
_____
_____

Did you feel that your health has improved? Did you feel more energetic?
_____
_____

REVIEWS OF Exercise:

Duration:

Calories Burned:

Rating:
☆☆☆☆☆

DATE: _____

TODAY'S INTENTION:
_____
_____
_____

M	T	W	T	F	S	S

MOOD:
- ❏ FABULOUS
- ❏ HAPPY
- ❏ SAD
- ❏ ANGRY

THINGS I AM GRATEFUL FOR TODAY:
_____
_____
_____

WHICH FORMS YOU HAVE EXERCISED FOR TODAY?
_____
_____

WHAT DO YOU LIKE/LEARN DURING TODAY'S EXERCISE?
_____
_____

WHAT WOULD YOU LIKE TO BE IMPROVED NEXT TIME?
_____
_____

DID YOU FEEL THAT YOUR HEALTH HAS IMPROVED? DID YOU FEEL MORE ENERGETIC?
_____
_____

REVIEWS OF EXERCISE:

DURATION:

CALORIES BURNED:

RATING:
☆☆☆☆☆

DATE: _____

| M | T | W | T | F | S | S |

Today's Intention:
_____
_____
_____

MOOD:
- ❑ Fabulous
- ❑ Happy
- ❑ Sad
- ❑ Angry

Things I am Grateful For Today:
_____
_____
_____

Which forms you have exercised for today?
_____
_____

What do you like/learn during today's exercise?
_____
_____

What would you like to be improved next time?
_____
_____

Did you feel that your health has improved? Did you feel more energetic?
_____
_____

REVIEWS OF EXERCISE:

DURATION:

CALORIES BURNED:

RATING:
☆☆☆☆☆

DATE: _____

| M | T | W | T | F | S | S |

Today's Intention:
_____
_____
_____

MOOD:
☐ Fabulous
☐ Happy
☐ Sad
☐ Angry

Things I am Grateful For Today:
_____
_____
_____

Which forms you have exercised for today?
_____
_____

What do you like/learn during today's exercise?
_____
_____

What would you like to be improved Next time?
_____
_____

Did you feel that your health has improved? Did you feel more energetic?
_____
_____

REVIEWS OF Exercise:

Duration:

Calories Burned:

Rating:
☆ ☆ ☆ ☆ ☆

Review

Review your experience with the past 10 days of your tai chi journey. Put down plans for the next 10 days.

NOT EVERYDAY IS SUNDAY. BUT YOU CAN MAKE IT A HAPPY DAY.

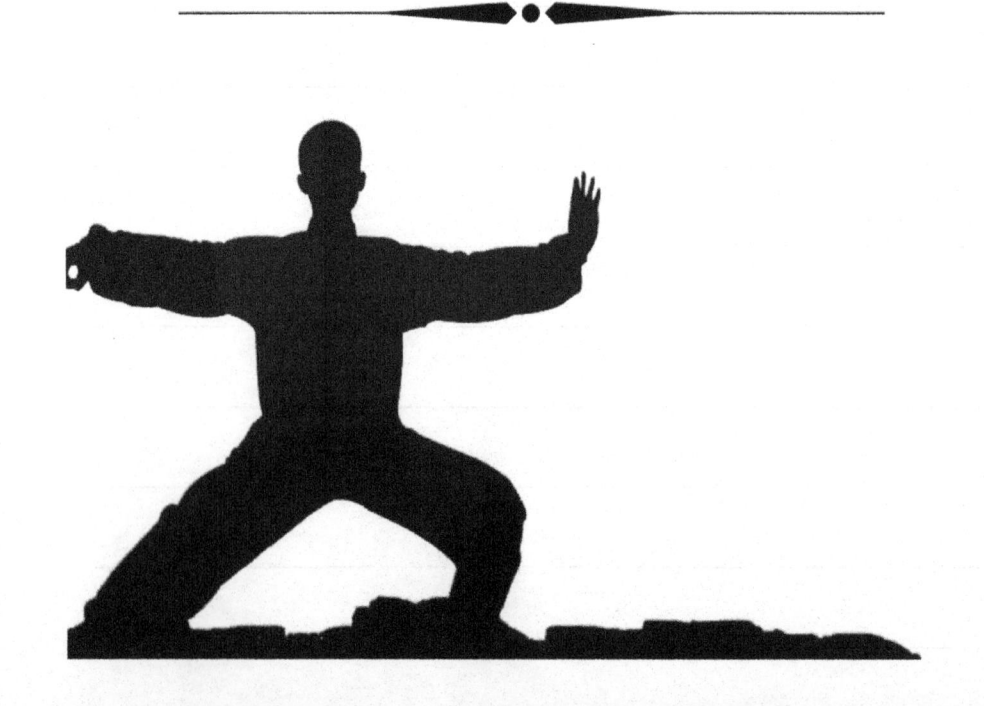

DATE: _____

| M | T | W | T | F | S | S |

TODAY'S INTENTION:
_____
_____
_____

MOOD:
- ❑ FABULOUS
- ❑ HAPPY
- ❑ SAD
- ❑ ANGRY

THINGS I AM GRATEFUL FOR TODAY:
_____
_____
_____

WHICH FORMS YOU HAVE EXERCISED FOR TODAY?
_____
_____

WHAT DO YOU LIKE/LEARN DURING TODAY'S EXERCISE?
_____
_____

WHAT WOULD YOU LIKE TO BE IMPROVED NEXT TIME?
_____
_____

DID YOU FEEL THAT YOUR HEALTH HAS IMPROVED? DID YOU FEEL MORE ENERGETIC?
_____
_____

REVIEWS OF EXERCISE:

DURATION:

CALORIES BURNED:

RATING:
☆☆☆☆☆

DATE: _____

| M | T | W | T | F | S | S |

TODAY'S INTENTION:
_____
_____
_____

MOOD:
❑ FABULOUS
❑ HAPPY
❑ SAD
❑ ANGRY

THINGS I AM GRATEFUL FOR TODAY:
_____
_____
_____

WHICH FORMS YOU HAVE EXERCISED FOR TODAY?
_____
_____

WHAT DO YOU LIKE/LEARN DURING TODAY'S EXERCISE?
_____
_____

WHAT WOULD YOU LIKE TO BE IMPROVED NEXT TIME?
_____
_____

DID YOU FEEL THAT YOUR HEALTH HAS IMPROVED? DID YOU FEEL MORE ENERGETIC?
_____
_____

REVIEWS OF EXERCISE:

DURATION:

CALORIES BURNED:

RATING:
☆☆☆☆☆

DATE: _____

| M | T | W | T | F | S | S |

Today's Intention:
_____
_____
_____

Mood:
- ❑ Fabulous
- ❑ Happy
- ❑ Sad
- ❑ Angry

Things I am Grateful For Today:
_____
_____
_____

Which forms you have exercised for today?
_____
_____

What do you like/learn during today's exercise?
_____
_____

What would you like to be improved next time?
_____
_____

Did you feel that your health has improved? Did you feel more energetic?
_____

Reviews of Exercise:

Duration:

Calories Burned:

Rating:
☆☆☆☆☆

DATE: _____

M	T	W	T	F	S	S

Today's Intention:
_____
_____
_____

MOOD:
- ❏ Fabulous
- ❏ Happy
- ❏ Sad
- ❏ Angry

Things I am Grateful For Today:
_____
_____
_____

Which forms you have exercised for today?
_____
_____

What do you like/learn during today's exercise?
_____
_____

What would you like to be improved Next time?
_____
_____

Did you feel that your health has improved? Did you feel more energetic?
_____
_____

Reviews of Exercise:

Duration:

Calories Burned:

Rating: ☆☆☆☆☆

DATE: _____

M	T	W	T	F	S	S

Today's Intention:
_____
_____
_____

MOOD:
- ❑ Fabulous
- ❑ Happy
- ❑ Sad
- ❑ Angry

Things I am Grateful For Today:
_____
_____
_____

Which forms you have exercised for today?
_____
_____

What do you like/learn during today's exercise?
_____
_____

What would you like to be improved Next time?
_____
_____

Did you feel that your health has improved? Did you feel more energetic?
_____
_____

REVIEWS OF Exercise:

Duration:

Calories Burned:

Rating:
☆☆☆☆☆

DATE: _____

| M | T | W | T | F | S | S |

Today's Intention:
_____
_____
_____

MOOD:
- ❑ Fabulous
- ❑ Happy
- ❑ Sad
- ❑ Angry

Things I am Grateful For Today:
_____
_____
_____

Which forms you have exercised for today?
_____
_____

What do you like/learn during today's exercise?
_____
_____

What would you like to be improved Next time?
_____
_____

Did you feel that your health has improved? Did you feel more energetic?
_____
_____

REVIEWS OF EXERCISE:

DURATION:

CALORIES BURNED:

RATING:
☆☆☆☆☆

DATE: _____

| M | T | W | T | F | S | S |

Today's Intention:
_____
_____
_____

MOOD:
- ❑ Fabulous
- ❑ Happy
- ❑ Sad
- ❑ Angry

Things I am Grateful For Today:
_____
_____
_____

Which forms you have exercised for today?
_____
_____

What do you like/learn during today's exercise?
_____
_____

What would you like to be improved Next time?
_____
_____

Did you feel that your health has improved? Did you feel more energetic?
_____
_____

Reviews of Exercise:

Duration:

Calories Burned:

Rating:
☆☆☆☆☆

DATE: _____

| M | T | W | T | F | S | S |

Today's Intention:
_____
_____
_____

MOOD:
- ❏ Fabulous
- ❏ Happy
- ❏ Sad
- ❏ Angry

Things I am Grateful For Today:
_____
_____
_____

Which forms you have exercised for today?
_____
_____

What do you like/learn during today's exercise?
_____
_____

What would you like to be improved Next time?
_____
_____

Did you feel that your health has improved? Did you feel more energetic?
_____
_____

REVIEWS OF EXERCISE:

Duration:

Calories Burned:

Rating:
☆☆☆☆☆

DATE: _____

| M | T | W | T | F | S | S |

Today's Intention:
_____
_____
_____

MOOD:
- ❏ Fabulous
- ❏ Happy
- ❏ Sad
- ❏ Angry

Things I am Grateful For Today:
_____
_____
_____

Which forms you have exercised for today?
_____
_____

What do you like/learn during today's exercise?
_____
_____

What would you like to be improved Next time?
_____
_____

Did you feel that your health has improved? Did you feel more energetic?
_____
_____

Reviews of Exercise:

Duration:

Calories Burned:

Rating:
☆☆☆☆☆

DATE: _____

| M | T | W | T | F | S | S |

Today's Intention:
_____
_____
_____

MOOD:
- ❑ Fabulous
- ❑ Happy
- ❑ Sad
- ❑ Angry

Things I am Grateful For Today:
_____
_____
_____

Which forms you have exercised for today?
_____
_____

What do you like/learn during today's exercise?
_____
_____

What would you like to be improved Next time?
_____
_____

Did you feel that your health has improved? Did you feel more energetic?
_____
_____

REVIEWS OF Exercise:

Duration:

Calories Burned:

Rating:
☆☆☆☆☆

REVIEW

Review your experience with the past 10 days of your tai chi journey. Put down plans for the next 10 days.

_____
_____
_____
_____
_____
_____
_____
_____
_____
_____
_____
_____
_____
_____
_____
_____
_____
_____

Thankful people are more well-off than others.

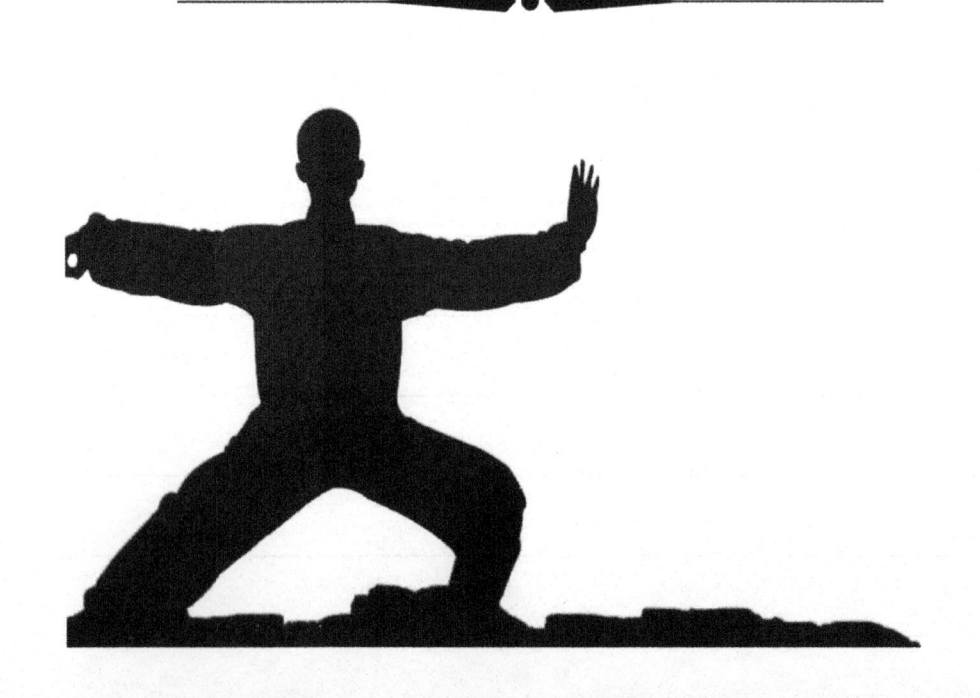

DATE: _____

| M | T | W | T | F | S | S |

TODAY'S INTENTION:
_____
_____
_____

MOOD:
- ❑ FABULOUS
- ❑ HAPPY
- ❑ SAD
- ❑ ANGRY

THINGS I AM GRATEFUL FOR TODAY:
_____
_____
_____

WHICH FORMS YOU HAVE EXERCISED FOR TODAY?
_____
_____

WHAT DO YOU LIKE/LEARN DURING TODAY'S EXERCISE?
_____
_____

WHAT WOULD YOU LIKE TO BE IMPROVED NEXT TIME?
_____
_____

DID YOU FEEL THAT YOUR HEALTH HAS IMPROVED? DID YOU FEEL MORE ENERGETIC?
_____
_____

REVIEWS OF EXERCISE:

DURATION:

CALORIES BURNED:

RATING:
☆☆☆☆☆

DATE: _____

| M | T | W | T | F | S | S |

Today's Intention:
_____
_____
_____

MOOD:
- ❏ Fabulous
- ❏ Happy
- ❏ Sad
- ❏ Angry

Things I am Grateful For Today:
_____
_____
_____

Which forms you have exercised for today?
_____
_____

What do you like/learn during today's exercise?
_____
_____

What would you like to be improved Next time?
_____
_____

Did you feel that your health has improved? Did you feel more energetic?
_____

Reviews of Exercise:

Duration:

Calories Burned:

Rating:
☆☆☆☆☆

DATE: _____

| M | T | W | T | F | S | S |

TODAY'S INTENTION:
_____
_____
_____

MOOD:
- ❏ FABULOUS
- ❏ HAPPY
- ❏ SAD
- ❏ ANGRY

THINGS I AM GRATEFUL FOR TODAY:
_____
_____
_____

WHICH FORMS YOU HAVE EXERCISED FOR TODAY?
_____
_____

WHAT DO YOU LIKE/LEARN DURING TODAY'S EXERCISE?
_____
_____

WHAT WOULD YOU LIKE TO BE IMPROVED NEXT TIME?
_____
_____

DID YOU FEEL THAT YOUR HEALTH HAS IMPROVED? DID YOU FEEL MORE ENERGETIC?
_____
_____

REVIEWS OF EXERCISE:

DURATION:

CALORIES BURNED:

RATING:
☆☆☆☆☆

DATE: _____

| M | T | W | T | F | S | S |

Today's Intention:
_____
_____
_____

MOOD:
- ❏ Fabulous
- ❏ Happy
- ❏ Sad
- ❏ Angry

Things I am Grateful For Today:
_____
_____
_____

Which forms you have exercised for today?
_____
_____

What do you like/learn during today's exercise?
_____
_____

What would you like to be improved Next time?
_____
_____

Did you feel that your health has improved? Did you feel more energetic?
_____
_____

Reviews of Exercise:

Duration:

Calories Burned:

Rating:
☆☆☆☆☆

DATE: _____

M	T	W	T	F	S	S

Today's Intention:
_____
_____
_____

MOOD:
- ❏ Fabulous
- ❏ Happy
- ❏ Sad
- ❏ Angry

Things I am Grateful For Today:
_____
_____
_____

Which forms you have exercised for today?
_____
_____

What do you like/learn during today's exercise?
_____
_____

What would you like to be improved Next time?
_____
_____

Did you feel that your health has improved? Did you feel more energetic?
_____
_____

Reviews of Exercise:

Duration:

Calories Burned:

Rating:
☆☆☆☆☆

DATE: _____

| M | T | W | T | F | S | S |

Today's Intention:
_____
_____
_____

MOOD:
- ❑ Fabulous
- ❑ Happy
- ❑ Sad
- ❑ Angry

Things I am Grateful For Today:
_____
_____
_____

Which forms you have exercised for today?
_____
_____

What do you like/learn during today's exercise?
_____
_____

What would you like to be improved Next time?
_____
_____

Did you feel that your health has improved? Did you feel more energetic?
_____
_____

Reviews of Exercise:

Duration:

Calories Burned:

Rating:
☆☆☆☆☆

DATE: _____

| M | T | W | T | F | S | S |

TODAY'S INTENTION:
_____
_____
_____

MOOD:
- ❑ FABULOUS
- ❑ HAPPY
- ❑ SAD
- ❑ ANGRY

THINGS I AM GRATEFUL FOR TODAY:
_____
_____
_____

WHICH FORMS YOU HAVE EXERCISED FOR TODAY?
_____
_____

WHAT DO YOU LIKE/LEARN DURING TODAY'S EXERCISE?
_____
_____

WHAT WOULD YOU LIKE TO BE IMPROVED NEXT TIME?
_____
_____

DID YOU FEEL THAT YOUR HEALTH HAS IMPROVED? DID YOU FEEL MORE ENERGETIC?
_____
_____

REVIEWS OF EXERCISE:

DURATION:

CALORIES BURNED:

RATING:
☆☆☆☆☆

DATE: _____

| M | T | W | T | F | S | S |

Today's Intention:
_____
_____
_____

Mood:
- ❏ Fabulous
- ❏ Happy
- ❏ Sad
- ❏ Angry

Things I am Grateful For Today:
_____
_____
_____

Which forms you have exercised for today?
_____
_____

What do you like/learn during today's exercise?
_____
_____

What would you like to be improved Next time?
_____
_____

Did you feel that your health has improved? Did you feel more energetic?
_____
_____

Reviews of Exercise:

Duration:

Calories Burned:

Rating:
★★★★☆

DATE: _____

| M | T | W | T | F | S | S |

Today's Intention:
_____
_____
_____

Mood:
- ❏ Fabulous
- ❏ Happy
- ❏ Sad
- ❏ Angry

Things I am Grateful For Today:
_____
_____
_____

Which forms you have exercised for today?
_____
_____

What do you like/learn during today's exercise?
_____
_____

What would you like to be improved next time?
_____
_____

Did you feel that your health has improved? Did you feel more energetic?
_____
_____

Reviews of Exercise:

Duration:

Calories Burned:

Rating:
☆☆☆☆☆

DATE: _____

| M | T | W | T | F | S | S |

Today's Intention:
_____
_____
_____

MOOD:
- ❏ Fabulous
- ❏ Happy
- ❏ Sad
- ❏ Angry

Things I am Grateful For Today:
_____
_____
_____

Which forms you have exercised for today?
_____
_____

What do you like/learn during today's exercise?
_____
_____

What would you like to be improved Next time?
_____
_____

Did you feel that your health has improved? Did you feel more energetic?
_____
_____

REVIEWS OF Exercise:

Duration:

Calories Burned:

Rating:
☆☆☆☆☆

Review

Review your experience with the past 10 days of your tai chi journey. Put down plans for the next 10 days.

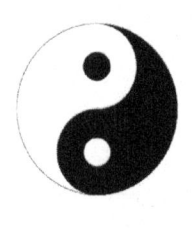

Gratitude opens your inside beauty.

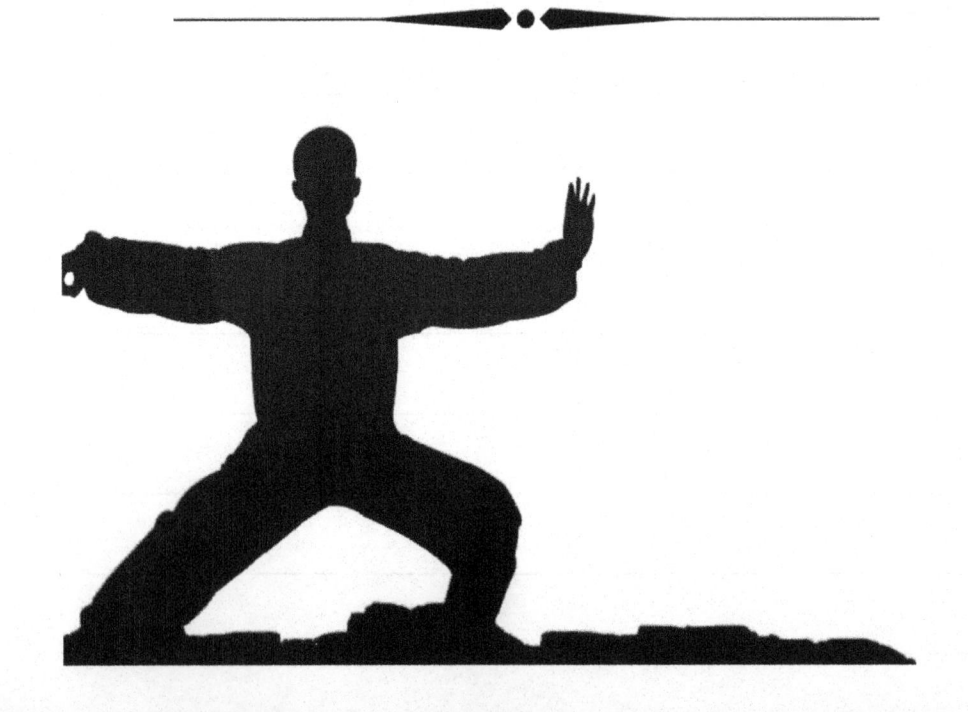

DATE: _____

| M | T | W | T | F | S | S |

TODAY'S INTENTION:
_____
_____
_____

MOOD:
- ❏ FABULOUS
- ❏ HAPPY
- ❏ SAD
- ❏ ANGRY

THINGS I AM GRATEFUL FOR TODAY:
_____
_____
_____

WHICH FORMS YOU HAVE EXERCISED FOR TODAY?
_____
_____

WHAT DO YOU LIKE/LEARN DURING TODAY'S EXERCISE?
_____
_____

WHAT WOULD YOU LIKE TO BE IMPROVED NEXT TIME?
_____
_____

DID YOU FEEL THAT YOUR HEALTH HAS IMPROVED? DID YOU FEEL MORE ENERGETIC?
_____
_____

REVIEWS OF EXERCISE:

DURATION:

CALORIES BURNED:

RATING:
☆☆☆☆☆

DATE: _____

| M | T | W | T | F | S | S |

Today's Intention:
_____
_____
_____

MOOD:
- ❏ Fabulous
- ❏ Happy
- ❏ Sad
- ❏ Angry

Things I am Grateful For Today:
_____
_____

Which forms you have exercised for today?
_____
_____

What do you like/learn during today's exercise?
_____
_____

What would you like to be improved Next time?
_____
_____

Did you feel that your health has improved? Did you feel more energetic?
_____
_____

Reviews of Exercise:

Duration:

Calories Burned:

Rating:
☆☆☆☆☆

DATE: _____

| M | T | W | T | F | S | S |

Today's Intention:
_____
_____
_____

MOOD:
- ❑ Fabulous
- ❑ Happy
- ❑ Sad
- ❑ Angry

Things I am Grateful For Today:
_____
_____
_____

Which forms you have exercised for today?
_____
_____

What do you like/learn during today's exercise?
_____
_____

What would you like to be improved Next time?
_____
_____

Did you feel that your health has improved? Did you feel more energetic?
_____
_____

REVIEWS OF EXERCISE:

DURATION:

CALORIES BURNED:

RATING:
☆☆☆☆☆

DATE: _____

| M | T | W | T | F | S | S |

Today's Intention:
_____
_____
_____

MOOD:
- ❏ Fabulous
- ❏ Happy
- ❏ Sad
- ❏ Angry

Things I am Grateful For Today:
_____
_____
_____

Which forms you have exercised for today?
_____
_____

What do you like/learn during today's exercise?
_____
_____

What would you like to be improved Next time?
_____
_____

Did you feel that your health has improved? Did you feel more energetic?
_____
_____

REVIEWS OF Exercise:

Duration:

Calories Burned:

Rating:
☆☆☆☆☆

DATE: _____

| M | T | W | T | F | S | S |

Today's Intention:
_____
_____
_____

MOOD:
- ❏ Fabulous
- ❏ Happy
- ❏ Sad
- ❏ Angry

Things I am Grateful For Today:
_____
_____
_____

Which forms you have exercised for today?
_____
_____

What do you like/learn during today's exercise?
_____
_____

What would you like to be improved Next time?
_____
_____

Did you feel that your health has improved? Did you feel more energetic?
_____
_____

Reviews of Exercise:

Duration:

Calories Burned:

Rating: ☆☆☆☆☆

DATE: _____

| M | T | W | T | F | S | S |

TODAY'S INTENTION:
_____
_____
_____
_____

MOOD:
- ❏ FABULOUS
- ❏ HAPPY
- ❏ SAD
- ❏ ANGRY

THINGS I AM GRATEFUL FOR TODAY:
_____
_____
_____

WHICH FORMS YOU HAVE EXERCISED FOR TODAY?
_____
_____

WHAT DO YOU LIKE/LEARN DURING TODAY'S EXERCISE?
_____
_____

WHAT WOULD YOU LIKE TO BE IMPROVED NEXT TIME?
_____
_____

DID YOU FEEL THAT YOUR HEALTH HAS IMPROVED? DID YOU FEEL MORE ENERGETIC?
_____
_____

REVIEWS OF EXERCISE:

DURATION:

CALORIES BURNED:

RATING:
☆☆☆☆☆

DATE: _____

| M | T | W | T | F | S | S |

Today's Intention:
_____
_____
_____

MOOD:
- ❏ Fabulous
- ❏ Happy
- ❏ Sad
- ❏ Angry

Things I am Grateful For Today:
_____
_____
_____

Which forms you have exercised for today?
_____
_____

What do you like/learn during today's exercise?
_____
_____

What would you like to be improved Next time?
_____
_____

Did you feel that your health has improved? Did you feel more energetic?
_____
_____

Reviews of Exercise:

Duration:

Calories Burned:

Rating:
☆☆☆☆☆

DATE: _____

| M | T | W | T | F | S | S |

Today's Intention:
_____
_____
_____

MOOD:
- ❏ Fabulous
- ❏ Happy
- ❏ Sad
- ❏ Angry

Things I am Grateful For Today:
_____
_____
_____

Which forms you have exercised for today?
_____
_____

What do you like/learn during today's exercise?
_____
_____

What would you like to be improved Next time?
_____
_____

Did you feel that your health has improved? Did you feel more energetic?
_____
_____

Reviews of Exercise:

Duration:

Calories Burned:

Rating:
☆☆☆☆☆

DATE: _____

| M | T | W | T | F | S | S |

Today's Intention:
_____
_____
_____

MOOD:
- ❏ Fabulous
- ❏ Happy
- ❏ Sad
- ❏ Angry

Things I am Grateful For Today:
_____
_____
_____

Which forms you have exercised for today?
_____
_____

What do you like/learn during today's exercise?
_____
_____

What would you like to be improved next time?
_____
_____

Did you feel that your health has improved? Did you feel more energetic?
_____
_____

REVIEWS OF EXERCISE:

DURATION:

CALORIES BURNED:

RATING:
☆☆☆☆☆

DATE: _____

M	T	W	T	F	S	S

Today's Intention:
_____
_____
_____

Mood:
- ☐ Fabulous
- ☐ Happy
- ☐ Sad
- ☐ Angry

Things I am Grateful For Today:
_____
_____
_____

Which forms you have exercised for today?
_____
_____

What do you like/learn during today's exercise?
_____
_____

What would you like to be improved Next time?
_____
_____

Did you feel that your health has improved? Did you feel more energetic?
_____
_____

Reviews of Exercise:

Duration:

Calories Burned:

Rating:
☆☆☆☆☆

REVIEW

REVIEW YOUR EXPERIENCE WITH THE PAST 10 DAYS OF YOUR TAI CHI JOURNEY. PUT DOWN PLANS FOR THE NEXT 10 DAYS.

DISCLAIMER:

THE AUTHORS AND PUBLISHER OF THIS BOOK DISCLAIM ALL LIABILITY IN CONNECTION WITH THE USE OF THIS BOOK AND DISAVOW ALL KNOWLEDGE OF PERSONAL DETAILS WRITTEN INTO THIS AFTER PUBLICATION. THE CONTENTS OF THIS BOOK ARE SOLELY FOR THE PURCHASER'S PRIVATE USE AND WILL BE TREATED AS SUCH UNDER THE JURISDICTION OF THE UNITED STATES OF AMERICA, AND UNDER RECOGNIZED INTERNATIONAL PUBLISHING LAWS. ALL PERSONS CONCERNED ABOUT MEDICAL SYMPTOMS OR THE POSSIBILITY OF DISEASE ARE ENCOURAGED TO SEEK PROFESSIONAL CARE FROM AN APPROPRIATE HEALTHCARE PROVIDER.

IN NO WAY IS THIS BOOK DESIGNED TO REPLACE, SUBSTITUTE, COUNTERMAND, OR CONFLICT WITH ADVICE GIVEN TO YOU BY YOUR PHYSICIAN, OR MENTAL HEALTH PROFESSIONAL. INFORMATION IN THIS BOOK IS OFFERED WITH NO GUARANTEES ON THE PART OF THE AUTHORS OR PUBLISHER. THIS BOOK IS NOT INTENDED AS A SUBSTITUTE FOR THE MEDICAL ADVICE OF PHYSICIANS. THE READER SHOULD REGULARLY CONSULT A PHYSICIAN IN MATTERS RELATING TO HIS/HER HEALTH AND PARTICULARLY WITH RESPECT TO ANY SYMPTOMS THAT MAY REQUIRE RECOMMENDATIONS OR SUGGESTIONS CONTAINED IN THIS BOOK.

SPECIALLY DESIGNED BY ZENWERKZ

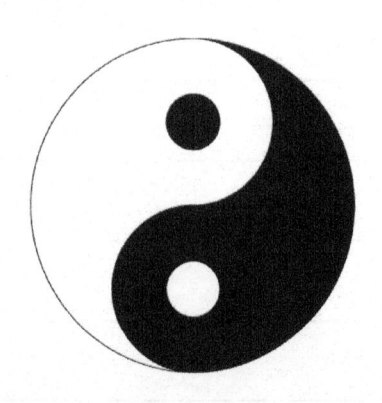

Made in the USA
Monee, IL
21 August 2025